NATURAL SOLUTION FOR ALLERGIC RHINITIS

Breathe Freely, Discovering Effective Natural Solutions To Combat Hay Fever

DR. JEREMY ALLEY

Disclaimer:

The information provided in this book, is intended for general informational purposes only and should not be considered as professional advice.

The author has made every effort to ensure the accuracy of the information presented. However, readers are advised to consult with a qualified healthcare professional before attempting any herbal remedies or making significant changes to their wellness routine. Individual health conditions vary, and what may be suitable for one person may not be appropriate for another.

It is important to note that the author is not in any endorsement deal, partnership, or affiliation with any organization, brand, or company mentioned in this book. Any references to specific products or services are based on the author's personal experience or general knowledge and do not imply an endorsement or promotion of those products or services.

Contents

CHAPTER ONE 16

UNDERSTANDING RHINITIS ALLERGIC............16

Types And Definition....................................16

Reasons And Initiators 17

Typical Symptoms..18

CHAPTER TWO 20

CLASSICAL MEDICATIONS 20

Synopsis Of Medications Traditionally Used.....20

Possible Adverse Reactions........................21

The Drawbacks Of Medicinal Methods 22

CHAPTER THREE 24

AN ALL-HOLISTIC TAKE ON ALLERGIC RHINITIS
....24

Overview Of Holistic Medicine......................24

Mind-Body Link..25

The Value Of An All-Encompassing Strategy....26

Natural Solutions For Allergy-Related Rhinitis..26

Combining Acupuncture With Allergic Rhinitis .27

Allergies And Local Honey 28

CHAPTER FOUR 32

RECOGNIZING ALLERGENS 32

Typical Allergens..32

Testing For Allergens 33

Techniques For Avoidance...............................33

Supplements And Dietary Adjustments 34

Herbal Treatments 35

Both Acupressure And Acupuncture................35

Yoga And Breathing Exercises........................36

CHAPTER FIVE..38

HABITAT AND NUTRITION................................38

Foods That Reduce Inflammation....................38

Items To Steer Clear Of 39

Supplements For Nutrition 40

CHAPTER SIX 42

HERBAL THERAPIES 42

An Overview Of Herbal Medicine.....................42

Herbs Particular To Allergic Rhinitis 43

Methodology And Application...........................44

CHAPTER SEVEN..46

AROMATHERAPY 46

Essential Oils For Allergy-Redness Syndrome ..46

Techniques Of Utilization 47

Establishing A Calm Ambience 47

CHAPTER EIGHT 50

HOMOPHATICAL MEDICATIONS 50

Overview Of Homeopathy..............................50

Typical Homeopathic Remedies.....................51

Individualized Methods...................................52

CHAPTER NINE...56

CLASSICAL MEDICINE METHODS 56

For Allergic Rhinitis, Acupuncture..................56

Allergies And Ayurveda...................................57

Chinese Traditional Medicine 57

CHAPTER TEN...60

ADVANCED LIFESTYLE CHANGES TO PREVENT ALLERGIES 60

Establishing A Salubrious Residence 61

Help For Making Your Home Allergy-Proof 62

Handling Allergies And Stress 62

CHAPTER ELEVEN...64

COMBINING MEDICAL TREATMENT WITH NATURAL REMEDIES 64

Speaking With Medical Experts 64

Having Conversations With Your Physician......65

Combined Methods 66

FINAL VERDICT......68

Recap Of Natural Treatments 69

Motivation To Lead A Healthier Lifestyle......69

Overview

Hay fever, often called allergic rhinitis, is a common allergic reaction that affects millions of individuals globally. Allergy rhinitis, which is characterized by symptoms including watery eyes, itching, congestion in the nose, and sneezing, can have a major negative effect on a person's quality of life. Although many doctors prescribe conventional pharmaceuticals to treat these symptoms, many people look for natural therapies as a complementary or alternative treatment option. This post will discuss some natural treatments for allergic rhinitis, their efficacy, and the significance of taking these options into account.

About This Book

The basic causes of allergic rhinitis must be understood before attempting any natural treatments. An immunological reaction to airborne allergens, including pollen, dust mites, animal dander, and mold spores, causes this illness. The immune system releases histamines in response to these allergens, which causes the well-known symptoms of allergic rhinitis.

It can be categorized as perennial—due to indoor allergens—or seasonal—occurring at particular seasons of the year when particular allergens are more common.

The Value of Natural Treatments

Natural treatments for allergic rhinitis are significant because they may reduce symptoms while having fewer adverse effects than some prescription drugs. Because natural therapies frequently address the underlying cause of allergies and help control the immune response instead of just treating symptoms, many people prefer them.

Furthermore, natural treatments for allergic rhinitis may provide a comprehensive strategy that addresses general health and well-being. Understanding the importance of natural therapies becomes crucial for people looking for a more integrated approach to controlling their allergic rhinitis as interest in alternative medicine develops.

Typical Home Treatments for Allergic Rhinitis

Many herbal therapies have demonstrated potential in mitigating the symptoms associated with allergic rhinitis. It is crucial to remember that each person will respond differently to these treatments, so speaking with a healthcare provider before using them in a treatment plan is advised. Typical natural therapies include the following:

Honey & Bee Pollen: It's thought that honey, particularly the raw, locally sourced types, contains trace amounts of local pollen.

Honey consumption may aid in the immune system's desensitization to these allergens. Some people think that bee pollen, which has anti-inflammatory qualities, can treat allergic rhinitis naturally.

Foods High in Quercetin: Quercetin is a naturally occurring antihistamine that can be found in some foods, such as berries, onions, and apples. It may help lessen allergic symptoms. Consuming foods high in quercetin may have anti-inflammatory and antihistaminic properties.

Saline Solution Nasal Irrigation: By flushing allergens and irritants from the nasal passages, saline solution nasal irrigation helps reduce congestion and enhance nasal airflow. Most people who perform this practice use a neti pot or saline nasal spray.

Butterbur Extract: The herb known as butterbur, which is indigenous to Europe, has been researched for its ability to lessen the symptoms of allergic rhinitis. Because butterbur extract doesn't include pyrrolizidine alkaloids (PA), it might be able to relieve allergic reactions such as congestion in the nose.

Probiotics: Immune system regulation is influenced by the balance of gut flora.

Probiotics, which are present in fermented foods like kimchi and yogurt, may influence the immune system and lessen allergy symptoms by supporting healthy gut flora.

Herbal Teas: Some herbal teas, such as peppermint and chamomile, have calming and anti-inflammatory qualities.

Sipping these teas can help improve respiratory health in general and alleviate symptoms of allergic rhinitis.

For those looking for alternatives to prescription drugs, natural treatments for allergic rhinitis provide a variety of choices.

Even while these treatments might help some people, it's important to use caution when using them and speak with a healthcare provider, especially if you have serious allergies or underlying medical issues.

A thorough allergy treatment strategy that incorporates natural remedies can help with both symptom control and general well-being.

CHAPTER ONE

UNDERSTANDING RHINITIS ALLERGIC

A common illness called allergic rhinitis is characterized by inflammation of the nasal passages brought on by allergens. This illness, commonly known as hay fever, can seriously lower someone's quality of life. It is essential to comprehend the different facets of allergic rhinitis, such as its forms, definition, causes, and symptoms, to effectively manage and alleviate symptoms.

Types And Definition

An allergic reaction to allergens can result in allergic rhinitis, a persistent inflammatory condition of the nasal mucosa. Seasonal and perennial allergic rhinitis are the two main varieties. As the name implies, seasonal allergic rhinitis happens during particular seasons when certain plants discharge their pollen. Conversely, mold, dust mites, and pet dander are common indoor allergens that cause perennial allergic rhinitis, which lasts all year.

Reasons And Initiators

The body's immune system overreacting to innocuous molecules in the environment, known as allergens, is the main cause of allergic rhinitis.

Pollen from grasses, trees, and weeds is a common outdoor allergen; dust mites, pet hair, mold spores, and cockroach droppings are common indoor allergies.

The symptoms of allergic rhinitis can be brought on by exposure to certain allergens, which can cause the release of histamines and other substances.

Effective therapy for allergic rhinitis requires the identification of certain triggers.

Environmental elements that can aggravate symptoms include air pollution and weather variations. Furthermore, in vulnerable individuals, specific occupational exposures may have a role in the onset or exacerbation of allergic rhinitis.

Typical Symptoms

There is a wide range of symptoms associated with allergic rhinitis, such as runny nose, itchy or watery eyes, sneezing, and itching in the throat and nose. The quality of one's sleep, everyday activities, and general well-being can all be severely impacted by these symptoms.

To guarantee a precise diagnosis and suitable treatment, it's critical to distinguish allergic rhinitis from other respiratory disorders, such as viral infections or non-allergic rhinitis.

The allergic march is a phenomenon that people with allergic rhinitis may encounter.

If left untreated, allergic rhinitis can lead to other allergic disorders including asthma or eczema. Early diagnosis and treatment of allergic rhinitis can help avoid the emergence of associated problems.

Gaining a basis for managing and mitigating the effects of this frequent allergic ailment involves comprehending the basic features of allergic rhinitis, including its diagnosis, types, causes, and common symptoms.

CHAPTER TWO

CLASSICAL MEDICATIONS

Hay fever, sometimes referred to as allergic rhinitis, is a common illness marked by inflammation of the nasal passages as a result of an allergic reaction.

A growing number of people are interested in natural treatments for allergic rhinitis, even though conventional treatments frequently involve pharmaceutical interventions.

These substitutes seek to alleviate symptoms without the possible adverse reactions connected to some prescription drugs.

Synopsis Of Medications Traditionally Used

The three main drugs used to treat allergic rhinitis traditionally are corticosteroids, decongestants, and antihistamines.

The effects of histamine, a substance generated during an allergic reaction, are countered by antihistamines like loratadine and cetirizine. Decongestants that constrict blood vessels, such as pseudoephedrine, aid in the relief of nasal congestion.

Corticosteroids lessen nasal channel irritation; they are available as oral or nasal sprays. Although some drugs can be useful in treating symptoms, their possible adverse effects may make them unsuitable for everyone.

Possible Adverse Reactions

Conventional treatments for allergic rhinitis might have several negative effects, even though they are effective.

Symptoms of antihistamines include dry mouth, impaired vision, and sleepiness

. Decongestants may cause agitation, sleeplessness, and elevated blood pressure.

Nasal discomfort and nosebleeds may occur from using corticosteroid nasal sprays for an extended period.

Oral corticosteroids may also cause more severe adverse effects including weight gain, osteoporosis, and an elevated risk of infections. People may turn to natural therapies that provide relief without the negative consequences of pharmaceutical techniques as a result of these possible adverse effects.

The Drawbacks Of Medicinal Methods

Conventional drugs have various drawbacks even though they are successful in managing the symptoms of allergic rhinitis.

Some people may not get enough relief from these drugs or may have negative side effects.

In addition, prolonged usage of specific medications might not be recommended because of possible health hazards. Concerns exist over these drugs' effects on the immune system as well.

As a result, there is growing interest in investigating complementary and alternative medicine options that target allergic rhinitis holistically and seek to relieve symptoms without the possible side effects of medication.

CHAPTER THREE

AN ALL-HOLISTIC TAKE ON ALLERGIC RHINITIS

Hay fever, sometimes referred to as allergic rhinitis, is a disorder marked by inflammation of the nasal passages brought on by an allergic reaction to airborne allergens. While antihistamines and nasal corticosteroids, two common medical therapies, can help manage symptoms, many people look for natural and alternative solutions. The holistic technique is one such strategy that takes into account how the environment, body, and mind are interconnected.

Overview Of Holistic Medicine

The goal of holistic healing is to treat the full person, taking into account not just the physical symptoms but also the mental, emotional, and spiritual well-being of the patient. When it comes to treating allergic rhinitis, holistic therapy entails taking stress management, lifestyle modifications, and using natural therapies to reduce symptoms. This method acknowledges the interdependence of the body's systems and how imbalances in one can impact general health.

Mind-Body Link

A key component of the holistic approach to treating allergic rhinitis is the mind-body link. It is well-recognized that stress can worsen allergy symptoms.

To assist in reducing stress, try mindfulness, meditation, and deep breathing exercises.

The goals of mind-body therapies are to increase body awareness of allergies and facilitate relaxation. People who are in a pleasant mental state may see a decrease in the frequency and intensity of their allergic rhinitis symptoms.

The Value Of An All-Encompassing Strategy

An all-encompassing strategy for treating allergic rhinitis entails taking care of a person's life to enhance general well-being. This covers environmental influences, physical exercise, and food choices. A well-nourished immune system is more resilient to allergens, and a well-balanced diet high in vitamins and minerals can help achieve this. Regular exercise can also strengthen the immune system and lower inflammation, which may help to lessen the symptoms of allergic rhinitis.

Natural Solutions For Allergy-Related Rhinitis

For millennia, traditional medical systems have employed herbs to treat allergic symptoms. For instance, butterbur has demonstrated potential in lowering the frequency and intensity of symptoms associated with allergic rhinitis. Apples and onions contain quercetin, another natural chemical with anti-inflammatory qualities that may aid with allergy management. To make sure herbal medicines don't worsen pre-existing medical disorders or interfere with other prescriptions, it is crucial to speak with a healthcare provider before introducing them into a treatment plan.

Combining Acupuncture With Allergic Rhinitis

To promote the flow of energy through the body, tiny needles were inserted into certain locations during the ancient Chinese medicinal practice of acupuncture. According to certain research, acupuncture may be useful in alleviating the symptoms of allergic rhinitis by influencing the immune system and lowering inflammation. Some people get relief with acupuncture, although further research is necessary to fully understand the mechanics and effectiveness of this alternative medicine in treating allergic rhinitis.

Gut Health with Probiotics

The immune system depends on the gut microbiome, and allergies may be caused by bacterial imbalances in the stomach. Beneficial bacteria called probiotics may help control the immune system and lessen allergic irritation. The symptoms of allergic rhinitis may be alleviated by including probiotic-rich foods like yogurt, kefir, and sauerkraut in the diet or by taking probiotic supplements. Probiotic reactions differ from person to person, therefore speaking with a healthcare professional is advised.

Allergies And Local Honey

Because of the immunotherapy idea, local honey is widely promoted as a natural treatment for allergic rhinitis. The theory is that by ingesting modest amounts of local honey, which contains local pollen, the immune system may become less sensitive to certain allergens.

Although some individuals assert that this method relieves their rhinitis, there is little scientific proof to back up the effectiveness of local honey in treating the condition.

Furthermore, people with pollen allergies should exercise caution because raw honey might cause negative reactions.

A comprehensive strategy for treating allergic rhinitis includes a wide range of dietary adjustments, home cures, and complementary therapies that target the root causes of allergy symptoms.

These methods can supplement current procedures and provide people with a more thorough and individualized approach to managing their allergic rhinitis, even though they might not completely replace traditional medical therapies.

To develop a customized plan that addresses their unique needs and guarantees the safe incorporation of natural treatments into their overall allergy management strategy, people must collaborate with healthcare specialists.

CHAPTER FOUR

RECOGNIZING ALLERGENS

For effective therapy, determining which specific allergens cause allergic rhinitis is essential. Airborne pollutants like pollen, dust mites, mold spores, pet dander, and certain foods can cause allergic rhinitis. Identifying the particular allergens that a person is affected by is the first step in using customized natural therapies.

Typical Allergens

Allergies to several common allergens can cause allergic rhinitis. Outside triggers include grasses, trees, and weeds; indoor allergens include mold, dust mites, and pet dander. Furthermore, for those who are vulnerable, specific foods such as dairy, shellfish, and nuts might cause allergic reactions. Identifying these common allergens is crucial to creating a thorough natural treatment regimen.

Testing For Allergens

To pinpoint particular triggers that lead to allergic rhinitis, allergen testing is a useful diagnostic technique. Allergens can be identified with the use of blood tests like the IgE antibody test and skin prick testing. In skin prick testing, allergens are applied topically in tiny doses, and any resulting allergic reactions are monitored. Blood tests quantify the amounts of particular antibodies generated in reaction to allergens. Precise allergy testing allows people to customize their natural treatment regimen according to recognized triggers.

Techniques For Avoidance

After allergies are identified, it is critical to put avoidance tactics into practice. Using air purifiers, closing windows, and remaining inside during pollen-heavy seasons can all help reduce exposure to outdoor allergens like pollen. Using allergen-proof mattresses and pillow covers, keeping humidity levels low, and routine cleaning can all help reduce indoor allergens like mold and dust mites. Pet owners may need to use air purifiers and keep their pets out of bedrooms to reduce exposure. Dietary adjustments could also be required to stay away from foods that provoke allergies.

Supplements And Dietary Adjustments

A few dietary adjustments and supplements may be able to relieve allergic rhinitis naturally. Fruits and vegetables naturally contain quercetin, an antioxidant with anti-inflammatory qualities that may help reduce symptoms. Flaxseed and fish oil are rich sources of omega-3 fatty acids, which have anti-inflammatory properties and may help lessen allergic symptoms. Fermented foods and supplements containing probiotics can improve gut health and regulate the immune system, which may help reduce allergic reactions.

Herbal Treatments

For decades, herbal medicines have been utilized to treat a wide range of health conditions, including allergic rhinitis. Derived from Petasites hybridus, butterbur has demonstrated the potential to mitigate symptoms associated with allergies. When consumed as a tea or as a supplement, stinging nettle may have anti-inflammatory properties. Herbs like eucalyptus or chamomile are frequently added to saline solutions for nasal irrigation, which helps open up nasal passages and lessen symptoms.

Both Acupressure And Acupuncture

The potential of alternative therapies like acupuncture and acupressure to treat the symptoms of allergic rhinitis has drawn interest. The goal of acupuncture is to balance the flow of qi by inserting tiny needles into particular body locations. The same sites are compressed in acupressure, a non-invasive therapy. Some people claim that by using these techniques, they can relieve their nasal congestion and other allergy symptoms, while research on their efficacy is still underway.

Yoga And Breathing Exercises

Including yoga in your regular practice and engaging in breathing exercises can help manage allergic rhinitis.

Diaphragmatic breathing is one of the deep breathing techniques that can help with relaxation and stress reduction, both of which can help with allergy symptoms.

Some yoga positions, especially those that focus on relaxation and deep breathing, may help clear the nasal passages and enhance respiratory health.

A variety of techniques are used in natural remedies for allergic rhinitis, including identification of allergens, avoidance tactics, dietary adjustments, herbal medicines, alternative therapy, and lifestyle modifications.

To develop a customized plan that takes into account the particular allergens and symptoms that are particular to their circumstances, people should speak with healthcare professionals. Combining different natural therapies can increase how well they relieve the symptoms of allergic rhinitis.

CHAPTER FIVE

HABITAT AND NUTRITION

Hay fever, sometimes referred to as allergic rhinitis, is characterized by inflammation of the nasal passages brought on by the immune system's overreaction to allergens in the air. Allergy rhinitis can be effectively treated using natural therapies, such as dietary and nutritional methods, in addition to pharmaceuticals, which are widely used to manage symptoms.

Foods That Reduce Inflammation

By including foods that are anti-inflammatory in your diet, you can lessen the general inflammation brought on by allergic rhinitis. Walnuts, flaxseeds, and fatty fish (salmon, mackerel, and sardines) are examples of foods high in omega-3 fatty acids that have anti-inflammatory qualities. These meals might lessen the intensity of allergic responses and lessen the immunological response. Consuming foods strong in antioxidants, such as citrus fruits, berries, and leafy greens, can also strengthen the immune system and lessen the symptoms of allergies.

Items To Steer Clear Of

Avoiding some foods may help manage allergic rhinitis more successfully, as they can increase its symptoms.

Dairy items, especially cheese and full-fat milk, can increase mucus production, which may exacerbate nasal congestion.

Processed meals, which contain a lot of artificial ingredients and preservatives, might exacerbate preexisting conditions or cause allergic reactions.

Additionally, common allergens like nuts, shellfish, and gluten should be avoided by people who have allergic rhinitis because they might exacerbate allergic reactions and increase symptoms.

Supplements For Nutrition

By adding particular nutrients to your diet, you may strengthen your immune system and reduce the symptoms of allergic rhinitis. Because of its antioxidant qualities, vitamin C helps boost immunity and lessen inflammation.

Foods high in berries, onions, and apples contain quercetin, a flavonoid with anti-allergic qualities that may help treat allergic rhinitis. Probiotics are frequently present in fermented foods like kefir and yogurt.

They can support a healthy gut microbiome and may have an impact on allergic reactions and immune system performance.

 Furthermore, an herbal supplement called butterbur extract has demonstrated promise in easing the symptoms of allergic rhinitis;

nevertheless, you should always see a doctor before adding any new supplements to your regimen.

These home remedies for allergic rhinitis can be used in conjunction with conventional therapies when combined into a holistic approach. Before beginning a new supplement regimen or making big dietary changes, it is imperative to speak with a healthcare provider, particularly if you have underlying medical concerns or are currently taking other drugs.

CHAPTER SIX

HERBAL THERAPIES

Hay fever, sometimes referred to as allergic rhinitis, is a common ailment marked by inflammation of the nasal passages brought on by an allergic reaction to airborne particles. While nasal corticosteroids and antihistamines are common conventional treatments, many people look for complementary therapies, such as herbal medicines. Herbal treatments provide a safe and natural way to treat the symptoms of allergic rhinitis and have been utilized for millennia in many traditional medical systems worldwide.

An Overview Of Herbal Medicine

Phytotherapy, botanical medicine, and herbal medicine are terms used to describe the use of plants and plant extracts to treat and prevent a variety of illnesses. The concept that plants have therapeutic qualities that can aid the body's natural healing processes is the basis of this age-old practice, which has been practiced for thousands of years. Certain herbs have become well-known in the context of allergic rhinitis due to their ability to reduce symptoms and offer comfort without the negative effects connected with some pharmaceutical treatments.

Herbs Particular To Allergic Rhinitis

Many herbs have been shown to have anti-inflammatory and antihistamine qualities, which makes them viable options for treating the symptoms of allergic rhinitis. One such plant that is well-known for its capacity to lessen nasal congestion and enhance airflow is butterbur (Petasites hybridus). Ginkgo biloba, another herb, has anti-inflammatory properties that may help reduce allergic symptoms. Apples and onions are good sources of quercetin, a flavonoid with antioxidant qualities that may also have anti-allergic effects. Furthermore, stinging nettle (Urtica dioica) is thought to lessen inflammation and may ease symptoms like itching and sneezing.

Methodology And Application

Herbal teas, tinctures, pills, or extracts are some of the dietary forms in which herbal therapies for allergic rhinitis can be eaten. For instance, butterbur is frequently sold as a supplement; to prevent negative effects, take the recommended quantity as directed.

Supplements containing ginkgo biloba are also commonly accessible, but it's important to speak with a healthcare provider to figure out the right dosage for your needs.

 Foods high in quercetin can be included in the diet, however, for individuals who prefer a more concentrated form, supplements are available. You can drink stinging nettle tea or take supplements.

Adhering to prescribed dosages and seeking advice from a healthcare professional is essential, particularly for people with pre-existing medical issues or those on additional medications.

Herbal treatments provide a holistic and all-natural way to treat the symptoms of allergic rhinitis. Although some people may get comfort from these cures, it's crucial to remember that different people respond differently to herbal medication.

To guarantee safety and effectiveness, it is advisable to speak with a healthcare provider before using herbal medicines in a treatment plan, just like with any other medical issue.

CHAPTER SEVEN

AROMATHERAPY

Aromatherapy is a comprehensive method that enhances both physical and mental well-being by utilizing the aromatic qualities of essential oils. The ability of this natural medicine to reduce allergic rhinitis symptoms has made it more well-liked.

Essential Oils For Allergy-Redness Syndrome

It has been discovered that several essential oils are useful in treating the symptoms of allergic rhinitis. Because of its anti-inflammatory qualities, peppermint oil helps facilitate better breathing and lessen nasal congestion. Because of its well-known decongestant properties, eucalyptus oil is useful for treating nasal stuffiness. Due to its relaxing qualities, lavender oil may help reduce the tension and anxiety that are frequently brought on by allergic reactions.

Techniques Of Utilization

There are several ways to apply essential oils to treat the symptoms of allergic rhinitis. Inhalation is one such technique. Breathing becomes easier and nasal congestion can be quickly relieved by inhaling the essential oil scent.

Another technique is topical application, which involves applying diluted essential oils to particular skin locations, like the temples or chest, to reduce symptoms.

Because essential oils are quite concentrated, it's critical to dilute them properly with carrier oil to avoid irritating the skin.

Establishing A Calm Ambience

Creating a calming atmosphere is crucial to optimizing the advantages of aromatherapy for the treatment of allergic rhinorrhea.

An aromatherapy diffuser can be used to spread the scent of essential oils across a space, resulting in a calming environment.

Selecting soothing fragrances, like chamomile or lavender, can ease tension and encourage relaxation, improving one's general sense of well-being.

In addition, reducing triggers that can worsen symptoms of allergic rhinitis requires keeping a clean and allergen-free living environment.

An all-natural and comprehensive method of treating the symptoms of allergic rhinitis is provided by aromatherapy, especially when using essential oils.

The carefully chosen oils, which include lavender, eucalyptus, and peppermint, have qualities that can ease nose congestion, lower stress levels, and improve respiratory health in general.

People with allergic rhinitis might investigate alternative options to conventional therapies for symptom alleviation by combining application techniques like inhalation and creating a calming atmosphere with diffusers.

Aromatherapy should be used carefully; be sure to dilute it appropriately and see a doctor if you have any worries or pre-existing medical disorders.

CHAPTER EIGHT

HOMOPHATICAL MEDICATIONS

Hay fever, also referred to as allergic rhinitis, is a disorder marked by inflammation of the nasal passages brought on by an allergic reaction.

Some people look for natural therapies to treat the underlying cause and reduce symptoms, even though conventional treatments frequently contain antihistamines and decongestants.

A comprehensive approach to treating allergic rhinitis is provided by homeopathic remedies, a subspecialty of alternative medicine. These natural cures are made from plants and are said to boost the body's natural healing processes.

Overview Of Homeopathy

Samuel Hahnemann created the alternative medical method known as homeopathy in the late 1700s. "Like cures like," which states that a chemical that produces symptoms in a healthy person may be used to treat comparable symptoms in an ill person, is the basic tenet of homeopathy. The goal of homeopathic medicines is to stimulate the body's natural healing mechanisms by using greatly diluted ingredients. Homeopathy aims to treat the underlying immune system imbalances that cause allergic reactions in the context of allergic rhinitis.

Typical Homeopathic Remedies

Several homeopathic treatments are frequently used to reduce allergic rhinitis symptoms. Onion-derived allium cepa is frequently suggested for people with runny noses and watery eyes. Table salt-based natrum muriaticum is recommended for people who sneeze and have nasal congestion. Sabadilla, which is made from a plant's seeds, is also used to treat symptoms including convulsive sneezing and ocular and nasal irritation. These treatments are chosen by the patient's unique constitution and particular symptoms.

Treatments for allergic rhinitis using homeopathy go beyond treating immediate symptoms. In homeopathy, constitutional prescribing is a customized method that takes into account the patient's general health, temperament, and particular symptoms. A qualified homeopath does a comprehensive evaluation to determine which constitutional cure best suits the individual's particular traits. This customized strategy seeks to improve the patient's general health, lessen the chance of subsequent allergic reactions, and relieve existing symptoms.

Individualized Methods

In the field of homeopathy, treating allergic rhinitis in a customized manner entails taking into account several variables that affect a person's health. An evaluation of the individual's physical, mental, and emotional health is part of this. Constitutional prescribing considers the patient's lifestyle, stress levels, and any underlying medical conditions in addition to their general constitution. Homeopathic practitioners seek to provide a holistic treatment plan that goes beyond symptom suppression by addressing these issues.

Depending on how each patient presents with their particular set of symptoms, individualized homeopathic therapies may involve medicines like sulfur, pulsatilla, or nux vomica. People who have severe itching and persistent nasal congestion are frequently prescribed sulfur. Pulsatilla could be suggested for people who have erratic symptoms and a propensity for crying readily. Nux vomica, which comes from the strychnine tree's seeds, is used for people whose symptoms are made worse by stress, excessive labor, or a sedentary lifestyle.

A natural and comprehensive strategy for treating allergic rhinitis is provided by homeopathic treatments.

Homeopathy seeks to activate the body's healing mechanisms and restore equilibrium, whether through customized constitutional prescribing or common therapies that target certain symptoms. While each person reacts differently to homeopathic therapies, some people find that using this alternative method improves their general well-being and relieves symptoms of allergic rhinitis.

CHAPTER NINE

CLASSICAL MEDICINE METHODS

Sneezing, stuffy or runny nose, and nasal congestion are some of the annoying symptoms of allergic rhinitis, also referred to as hay fever. Some people seek healing from ancient medical methods, even if contemporary medicine offers a variety of treatments. These alternative methods try to address the root causes of allergies and frequently center on holistic well-being.

For Allergic Rhinitis, Acupuncture

The traditional Chinese treatment of acupuncture, which involves inserting tiny needles into predetermined body sites, has grown in favor of a possible treatment for allergic rhinitis. Acupuncture proponents contend that the treatment improves general health by balancing the body's energy, or qi. Its efficacy in reducing allergy symptoms has been studied in some research, and the findings suggest that allergy sufferers may have advantages like less nasal congestion and an overall higher quality of life.

Allergies And Ayurveda

According to India's traditional medical system, Ayurveda, allergic rhinitis is caused by an imbalance in the body's doshas, especially Vata and Kapha. Herbal preparations and dietary and lifestyle modifications are common components of Ayurvedic allergy treatments. For the treatment of allergic rhinitis, holy basil, ginger, and turmeric are frequently utilized in Ayurveda. In addition, methods like using herbal teas and saline nasal irrigations may be suggested to control symptoms and strengthen the body's defenses.

Chinese Traditional Medicine

The term "traditional Chinese medicine" (TCM) refers to a variety of techniques, such as acupuncture, nutritional therapy, and herbal medicine. According to traditional Chinese medicine, allergic rhinitis is caused by disturbances in the body's meridians' flow and an imbalance in qi, or life force. TCM herbal medicines may consist of mixtures of several plants, such as magnolia and xanthium, which are thought to address the underlying reasons for allergies. A healthy and harmonious lifestyle is crucial for managing allergic rhinitis, so TCM practitioners may also suggest lifestyle changes.

Although these alternative approaches to treating allergic rhinitis are provided by traditional medicine, it is important to proceed cautiously and seek advice from medical professionals. Combining conventional therapies with scientifically proven medical interventions can offer a more all-encompassing method of treating allergic rhinitis and enhancing general health.

CHAPTER TEN

ADVANCED LIFESTYLE CHANGES TO PREVENT ALLERGIES

Hay fever, or allergic rhinitis, can have a serious negative effect on a person's quality of life. Adopting lifestyle modifications can be extremely important in preventing and controlling allergic reactions, even while drugs can offer some relief. Dietary changes are a key component, with an emphasis on an anti-inflammatory and immune-stimulating diet. Consuming antioxidant-rich meals including fruits, vegetables, and omega-3 fatty acids might strengthen the body's defenses against allergens.

Another way of living that can help prevent allergies is regular exercise. Exercise strengthens the immune system and lessens the intensity of allergic reactions. To reduce exposure to outdoor allergens, it's crucial to plan indoor activities during pollen-peaking seasons.

Establishing A Salubrious Residence

The management of allergic rhinitis is significantly influenced by our living environment. Creating a healthy living environment can greatly minimize allergy exposure. Sustaining indoor air quality is one important factor. Dust mites, pollen, and pet dander are just a few of the airborne allergens that can be successfully captured by using air purifiers with HEPA filters.

Furthermore, preventing the accumulation of indoor contaminants requires adequate ventilation. Reducing humidity and opening windows to let in fresh air can help prevent the growth of mold, a frequent allergy. Maintaining a clean living space can also be achieved by routine cleaning, particularly in areas where dust tends to collect.

Help For Making Your Home Allergy-Proof

Several steps are involved in allergy-proofing your house to reduce exposure to common allergens. Starting with the bedroom, where we spend a good deal of time, let's start. Dust mites can be kept out by using hypoallergenic bedding, such as mattress covers and pillowcases. Regularly washing bedding in hot water can also aid in the removal of allergies.

It's critical to address any allergy sources in the remaining areas of the house. Carpets and upholstery can be effectively cleaned of dust and pet dander by routinely using a vacuum cleaner fitted with a HEPA filter. Blinds are a better option than curtains when it comes to minimizing surfaces where allergens might collect.

Handling Allergies And Stress

Stress management is essential to preventing allergies because it has been shown that stress can exacerbate allergic reactions. Relaxation methods like yoga, meditation, and deep breathing can be incorporated into everyday routines to assist in reducing stress and, in turn, lessen the intensity of allergy symptoms.

Furthermore, the immune system depends heavily on getting enough sleep. Better control of allergic rhinitis and general well-being can result from maintaining a regular sleep pattern and a sleep environment free of allergens.

An all-encompassing strategy for treating allergic rhinitis entails dietary adjustments, regular exercise, and stress reduction.

Preventing and easing allergic reactions can be greatly aided by creating a healthy living environment through steps like upgrading indoor air quality and allergy-proofing the house.

CHAPTER ELEVEN

COMBINING MEDICAL TREATMENT WITH NATURAL REMEDIES

Hay fever, sometimes referred to as allergic rhinitis, is a common ailment marked by inflammation of the nasal passages brought on by an allergic reaction to airborne particles. Even though doctors frequently prescribe medications such as nasal corticosteroids and antihistamines, many people look for complementary and natural therapies to improve general health and reduce symptoms.

Speaking With Medical Experts

It is important to speak with medical professionals, such as an allergist or your primary care physician, before starting any natural therapy regimen. To create a safe and successful treatment plan, you must have a thorough grasp of your medical history as well as the particular causes of your allergic rhinitis. Natural treatments should be in line with your general health and medical needs, and healthcare specialists can give you specific advice and help in this regard.

Having Conversations With Your Physician

When thinking about using natural treatments for allergic rhinitis, it's important to be transparent with your physician. To prevent possible interactions, let your healthcare provider know about any current therapies you are taking, including any over-the-counter drugs or herbal supplements.

When natural therapies are used in conjunction with medical interventions, they are guaranteed to enhance general health rather than undermine it. Personalized treatment plans can be modified through routine check-ins with your physician, taking into account your unique response to both natural and medical approaches.

Combined Methods

In addition to prescription therapies for allergic rhinitis, several natural remedies can help relieve symptoms and enhance general quality of life.

Dietary Modifications: For some people, modifying their diets provides relief. Eating foods high in quercetin, like berries, onions, and apples, may lessen the severity of allergic reactions. Fish oil and flaxseed oil, which are rich sources of omega-3 fatty acids, may also have anti-inflammatory qualities.

Herbal Supplements: Studies have indicated that stinging nettle and butterbur supplements may help lessen the symptoms of allergic rhinitis. But before adding herbal supplements to your routine, it's important to speak with a doctor because they can have negative effects or interfere with other prescriptions.

Probiotics: Keeping the gut flora in a balanced, healthful state with probiotic supplements or fermented foods like yogurt might strengthen immunity and lessen the severity of allergic reactions.

Acupuncture: Acupuncture is an ancient Chinese therapy in which small needles are inserted into precise body sites. Some people claim that acupuncture relieves their symptoms. Acupuncture's effectiveness in treating allergic rhinitis is still being investigated, however, some research points to possible symptom relief.

Nasal irrigation: Rinsing the nasal passages with saline solutions or a neti pot will help clear out irritants and reduce congestion. This easy-to-use, low-cost method can help alleviate symptoms when combined with medical interventions.

It takes careful thought and cooperation with medical professionals to combine natural treatments with pharmaceutical treatments for allergic rhinitis. Although natural methods might provide further relief, they should be considered adjunctive rather than substitute treatments. Having a one-on-one consultation with a healthcare professional guarantees a customized and secure strategy, optimizing the possible advantages of both conventional and natural treatments for allergic rhinitis.

FINAL VERDICT

Herbal supplements, lifestyle changes, and alternative therapies like acupuncture are just a few of the many natural treatments available for allergic rhinitis. Even though many people find relief with these cures, it's important to speak with a healthcare provider before making any major modifications to one's treatment plan. Furthermore, a more comprehensive strategy that incorporates these natural therapies, identifies triggers and upholds a healthy lifestyle can help improve the management of allergic rhinitis symptoms.

Recap Of Natural Treatments

In conclusion, people with allergic rhinitis can investigate a range of natural treatments. These include probiotics, acupuncture, herbal supplements, nasal irrigation, and diet adjustments. These methods can work better when combined with lifestyle modifications including recognizing and avoiding triggers. To provide a comprehensive and individualized management plan, it is imperative to view natural therapies as an adjunct to traditional medical treatments.

Motivation To Lead A Healthier Lifestyle

Adopting a better lifestyle might be crucial in managing allergic rhinitis, in addition to specialized therapies. Frequent physical activity, sufficient sleep, and effective stress reduction enhance general health and may have a favorable effect on the immune system. Establishing a conducive atmosphere that reduces contact with allergens and prioritizes natural therapies can enable people to take charge of their symptoms of allergic rhinitis.